Emotions & Elation

The Journey of My Pregnancy

Banani Das Dhar

Woven Words Publishers OPC Pvt. Ltd.

Registered Office:

Vill: Raipur, P.O: Raipur Paschimbar,

Dist: Purba Midnapore, Pin: 721401,

West Bengal, India.

Branch Office(Operations): Hyderabad

www.wovenwordspublishers.com

Email: publish@wovenwordspublishers.com

First published by Half Baked Beans., 2018

Second publication by Woven Words Publishers OPC Pvt. Ltd., 2021

A MEMOIR

IMPRINT: WOVEN WORDS RED

ISBN 13: 978-81-949749-2-5

ISBN 10: 81-949749-2-5

Price: 250 INR

Printed and bound in India by Woven Words Publishers

Contents

Acknowledgements

I wish to thank my husband, Subhashish Dhar, for his immense love and support while sharing the tale of my pregnancy to the world. I dedicate this work to our son, Lakshya, for whom we are blessed. He has completed our family in ways he can never fathom.

Thanks to Mom (Mrs. Anjali Das) and Dad (Mr Basanta Das) for letting me live my dreams and for showering me with continuous love and care during pregnancy. Special thanks to my Mother-in-law (Mrs. Geeta Dhar) and my Father-in-law (Late Mr Prabir Kumar Dhar) for their blessings and love. Last but not the least, I thank my little brother, Nupur Das, for being my support system always.

I believe this labor of love is liked by my readers irrespective of gender and age.

Foreword

One is never totally prepared to be a parent... Never! You may read hundreds of books and articles but your journey is and will always be unique. Parenthood is truly as exciting as a roller coaster with loads of screaming thrown in for good measure.

But the good news is, that you not in it alone. Every parent around the world goes through the very same sentiments. Sharing one's true emotions and elations, only makes it that much more real and relatable.

This story of an urban couple, will resonate with all new parents and unlike most parenting tomes, this one also has the father sharing his emotions freely.

After all parenting is about both the mother and father as they bring up their child together and create memories to last for a lifetime.

Ruchita Dar Shah
Founder & CEO
First Moms Club

A Special Message

The journey towards becoming a mother is THE most incredible one for a woman, a blessing, a God's gift like none other! It's simply truly magical! Reminiscing my own journey more than 16 years ago, the memories are so vivid, every detail, every emotion permanently etched in my heart, always taking me back to a happy place in my life; thanking God for this most beautiful and wondrous experience.

It's indeed commendable that Banani has so keenly penned down her moments and experiences in this book. This is the closest one can get to reading a first-hand account and I am sure many will find emotions that they can relate to personally.

I have known Banani and Subhashish to be a vibrant, enthusiastic and involved couple teaming together fabulously to bring their bundle of joy into this world. Wishing them loads of love, luck, laughter and happiness and also many more fascinating memories in their lives ahead.

Dr Suman Singh
MBBS. MD.
Sr.Consultant(OB/GYN)
CloudNine Hospital
Jayanagar

The Essence of Motherhood

Motherhood is a bliss that has to be experienced to be believed. When those tiny, wrinkly pink fingers wrap themselves around yours, only then can you witness the miracle of life! Pregnancy is not just a stepping stone in the journey of womanhood, but a solid foundation for another life. Every woman goes through a plethora of emotions during this beautiful phase and mine was no different.

1

The Surprise

I went to the washroom in a frenzy to calm my anxious mind. I was nervous, with my hands trembling and legs shaking during the walk- a walk towards a new and a more responsible life. 'Calm Down, Calm Down. Whatever happens, happens for the best', I was frantically calming my inner self. I didn't know if I was shaking with fear or with excitement. 'No, I don't want to be too excited', I kept uttering to myself. Not sure what's going to happen next, my mind was plagued by tumultuous thoughts with so many emotions. I continued taking small steps towards the washroom. It was like taking an exam and waiting for the results. You want to know your fate and then not so much. Having failed in the past, being nervous was quite natural. Will this time be any different? I placed myself in God's hands and decided to accept whatever He decides for me.

My husband seemed quite unperturbed as if he was sure of the amazing serendipity. He didn't share my trepidation, the uneasiness and the anxiety. This made me a little angry but calmed me at the same time, if something like that was even possible. The missing periods which confused and made me hopeful at the same time seemed to give him more confidence. Otherwise, the only time he got to know about 'those days' was when I used to yell at him without any apparent reason. Hormonal changes, you see. Since we were so eager to welcome parenthood, my husband kept a track of my cycles better than a menstrual tracker. A promotion from a loving husband to a passionate father awaited him. And somehow, he sensed it!

It was the moment of truth. I asked him to be near the washroom. We were both ready to experience the thrill. I unwrapped the device and put a few drops of the fresh urine sample. The Dipstick didn't show any sign for the next 2-3 minutes and it was the longest wait of my life. I thought, 'maybe it just isn't meant to be'. I covered my face, saddened. I was not ready to face another failed attempt. He could sense my disappointment. Few seconds later, I peeped through my fingers that were covering my face. And just like that, a beatific smile spread across his lips and his face brightened.

'Honey! Look now.' I turned and he showed me the two dark-pink lines on the device. I was awestruck and my frozen face gave way to an expression of unbridled joy.

'This is finally happening', I muttered. My mind was engaged in short monologues with itself and I had goosebumps all over. This time I was shivering not because of any nervousness but because of the happiness we both were about to soak in. And this joy was nothing like anything we had experienced ever before. The moment that we were waiting for with bated breaths was finally in front of us. We embraced each other with tears of joy streaming down our cheeks. Subhashish squeezed me in his arms, almost lifting me high up in the air. 'I love you! I'm very happy today', he said feeling over the moon.

We could sense each other's happiness as we had both been waiting for this day to arrive. Being in a relationship with him for almost fifteen years now, our love was all-consuming, but this new development was going to take our bond to even greater heights.

We let the feeling sink in for a few moments.

'Don't you think it's time our parents should learn about this lovely surprise?' I asked.

'Yeah, let's dial in', he said.

I was a bit shy to disclose the news to my parents, since for them, I am still a kid who needs pampering and special

attention. For parents, we are never grown-ups. I decided to disclose this news to my brother first who is more like a friend to me. I knew he would transfer it to the right person.

'I am pregnant', I declared.

'What? Please let me sleep some more', his sleepy voice refused to believe me.

I almost screamed next time, 'Bhai, I'm pregnant. You are going to be a Mama (Maternal Uncle) soon.'

'What? What are you saying?', he was wide awake and even with the distance between us, I could sense his thrill.

'Where is Jij (Subhashish)?'

'He is making calls to his family', I said.

'Congrats to both of you, I'm so happy', he wished me and hung up the phone.

By then, I was sure that the news must have travelled to my parents' ears. And why not, it was THE breaking news after all!

After a few minutes, I mustered up some courage and shed my inhibitions to finally call my parents.

'Ma, did brother inform you?', I was curious to know their reaction.

'Yes, yes. We are so happy for both of you. May the choicest blessings be upon you both.' I could sense my mother choking up with joy. Her little girl was going to be a mother.

We talked for another couple of minutes and she transferred the call to my father. Similarly, we communicated the news to Subhashish's family. Heartfelt congratulations came next.

We were on cloud nine and we celebrated the whole day. Just being with each other, talking about the good old days we spent, our journey so far and of course the miraculous event of that day made us feel closer than ever before. A new life is being created, with our blood and flesh, can there be anything more beautiful?

A note from 'The soon-to-be-father':

Being married for three years, I was more aware of her cycles than she gave me credit for. And when she missed this one by a week, I was more than sure that we were pregnant. I was excited, a little scared and pretty unsure of how everything was going to change. But I kept my anxiety to myself and didn't push her to take any further tests. I know a lot was going through her mind too.

The day was not very far when she decided to take the home pregnancy test. I was nervous but tried to maintain a facade of calmness. Within minutes, we could see the two lines and if these home pregnancy test results are to be trusted, I was going to be a father. Hardly ever had I experienced so many emotions at the same time!

All I knew at this point was that there was a human being gestating in my wife's belly, but it was still an unknown feeling for me. In my head I was prodding the future. I'd provide for him, play with him, teach him, and some day he'd grow up and be an independent person. I remember being excited, but also thinking that my life would never be the same.

2

The First Heart-Beats

It was two days after our third marriage anniversary celebrations. I remember the day distinctly and vividly. We found ourselves waiting for our turn at the hospital. The place made me nervous, curious and excited-all at the same time. I had always been averse to hospitals, the smell of medicines, of syringes, etc. But I guess it was time for me to embrace these changes, changes that were going to be an important part of my life in the months to come.

The waiting hall was filled with big, rotund, potbellied women who were carrying their delicate darlings inside of them. The premises were clean and sterile. Unlike other multi-speciality hospitals, ours, thankfully, did not reek of medicines and spirits, the smell of which made me nauseous.

'You sit here and let me get you a glass of water', my husband politely offered. I adjusted myself in the corner of an orange sofa where other pregnant women had already couched themselves.

I ran a curious eye around and found all the mothers-to-be cheerful and their better halves taking good care of them. Amongst them were a few who were in their postpartum period, carrying their precious ones tucked in baby-holders.

'When is our turn?', I asked almost impatiently. No sooner did I ask than the attendant called for me.

'Mrs. Banani Das', she called. The announcement sounded like a courtier being called to a King's court. The thought made me smile.

'Yes, here', I got up and walked towards her along with my husband.

One of the nurses checked my weight and my blood pressure. We both then entered the all-white silent chamber, which had a very charming lady sitting in the middle. As it turned out, it was my gynaecologist, Dr. Suman Singh.

After having a rather serious conversation and delivering some medical advice, the doctor asked me to get the Early Pregnancy Scan and Blood Tests done. In addition, she congratulated us and asked me to come back after two days with the reports.

In the meantime, I was getting ready for the tests. The phobia of needles, blood, pain- basically any process that involved any kind of insertion into my body- made me feel nervous and nauseated.

'Sit down, please', the lab attendant asked.

Although I was seated in a properly-cushioned chair, my feet and palms were sweating and I felt a strong urge to urinate. However, I decided to hold it as my

urine was very 'precious' and was of prime interest to the laboratory assistant, I thought with a smile.
The lab attendant was getting his armoury ready, with the syringe, three cylindrical glass tubes, and a black elastic belt.

'It will hurt, right? Please do it slowly', I whispered my request to her. I hoped her reply would calm my nerves but the worst came out.

'It will pain madam, please don't scare', the attendant replied in her incorrect English.

My forehead started to drip with sweat as I tried to make sense of her reply. What was she trying to say? Did she ask me not to scare her or not to get scared myself? Reluctantly, I gave my left hand to the lab attendant who wrapped a black belt around my arm and immediately, I clasped my husband's palm, out of fear as much as for his support.

Within a few seconds, the lady drew fresh dark blood from my body in exactly the same fashion how mosquitoes suck blood, puncturing our skin. The long cylindrical tubes were filled with my blood. The worst was not over yet. I was asked to fill a small plastic jar with my urine. I did as asked and was happy to finally relieve my overstretched bladder.

Once the blood tests were done, I was asked to wait for the scan. I had to fill my details in a form before going out for the scan. Once we entered the scanning room, I was asked to lie down on a bed. I thought my ovaries would be scanned by rolling an iron shaped, gel-covered device over my belly. My thoughts were interrupted by the doctor who asked me to undress waist down. I complied with the instructions.

She started to roll the scanning device over my abdomen, but was unable to see my organs clearly. This is all because of those layers of cellulite, I grinned to myself.

The doctor sitting in front of the monitor asked me to bend and widen my legs and within no time she gently inserted a transducer, covered in a lot of gel through my vaginal orifice. My better half was asked to sit next to my bed where I was laid over a sheet of parchment paper. I was relieved to see him next to me as I badly needed his support.

I could feel the insertion of an inanimate object but my eyes drifted towards the monitor. The doctor was looking at the tiny creature living inside my cocoon and explained that the baby's senses were developed and it was aware of its surroundings. The baby was almost 0.6 mm in size, the size of a blueberry. Both mine and my husband's pupils were fixated on the monitor and we were amazed to hear our baby's first heartbeats. It was beating really fast as if to make us realize its existence. No sound in my entire life had sounded sweeter!

I turned towards my husband and saw those same joyful tears reflecting in his eyes as in mine. We were speechless at that momentous occasion and could only manage to look at each other. Those first heartbeats were enough to say a thousand words!

The lines that I remember:

My precious little baby
I have loved you from the start
You are a tiny miracle laying closely to my heart.

Each day I feel your presence,
Each day you quickly grow.
Each day your heart beats softly
As only I could know.

So I will keep this in a special
place And remember each
year through
of this every time of life, the months I carried you.

A note from 'The soon-to-be-father':

Soon after that, we were both eager to see a doctor and get the news confirmed. While we made an appointment with the doctor, I was thinking about a blood test. To my surprise, the doctor suggested a scan that would confirm the pregnancy.

Now, I've been to an ultrasound room before. But this time, it was different. We were not looking for any anomaly in the body, we were in search of a new life inside my wife. Inside the room, I was sweating even with the AC on. As the doctor scanned my wife's uterus, she stopped to show us a black dot on the screen and exclaimed: 'That's your baby!' It was just a dot. Nothing like what I imagined it to be. I had goosebumps all over and it was the most beautiful dot I had ever seen in my life.

Soon after, the doctor made us listen to a beating heart. When she told me those were the heartbeats of the fetus, my own heart skipped a beat. The scan was soon over, we came back from the hospital sure of the fact that we were soon going to be parents but unsure at the same time about how our lives were going to change thereafter.

3

Gloomy Mornings

Few days after the initial excitement had subsided, I found myself in a phase that I had heard of and dreaded. Welcome, Dear First Trimester! I found an appropriate nickname for it- The Period of Nausea and Bloating.

Trust me, I hated those mornings when I behaved like a slug. Personally, I'm quite an active person, be it the hectic business hours or the weekends to travel. This period made me forget who I used to be and I missed being 'me'. The pregnancy hormones were acting as antigens and my body, on the other hand, was trying harder every single day to cope up with them.

I was in such a state that even without any alcohol, I was in a state of perpetual hangover.

'I'm feeling pukish but not able to puke', my irritated voice almost shook my husband who was quietly following his morning ritual of reading the newspaper.

'Please eat something, you will feel better', he insisted.

'I don't feel like eating anything. I want to vomit', I replied. I stood by the sink, hoping that getting that bile out of my stomach would make me feel better. But Alas! the nausea continued even though I had vomited.

It was my turn to experience, first-hand, what most expectant mothers go through. The morning sickness left me so nauseated that I would remain in bed until eleven. It made me lethargic and I could not bring myself either to have breakfast or prepare it for my husband. It made me feel guilty but I just could not muster up the courage. I was getting overly sensitive to the smell of food. Just the thought of food would make me run to the washroom. Since I had to take care of my little baby, I would sometimes force-feed myself with a simple meal of rice and lentils. The trio of nausea, vomiting and acidity was making me miserable.

Not only the mornings but the evenings too were no less torturous, filled with attacks of nausea and vomiting and forever reminding me of their presence.

I was waiting for the time when I would finally be able to enjoy this glorious phase. I was getting restless and could not eat, sleep or work properly. My palate became bitter and I was losing my inner peace.

'Can you please get me a little salt?' I demanded just to get rid of that bitterness on my tongue. And Subhashish would run to the washroom with the jar of salt. No wonder pregnant women crave for sour things like raw mangoes.

I looked around for advice but none I received made me feel any better.

Most people I met used to tell me, 'Enjoy your pregnancy. It's such a beautiful experience.' But my heart said, 'Say that shit again and I will cut you!'

'It's normal', they would say. I decided to do something about it as I was not ready to be unhappy the whole day and went to see my doctor.

I had my list ready and bombarded the doctor with questions. I wondered if she thought if I had gone totally bonkers. Frankly, I didn't really care!

The doctor very gently laid my worries to rest and assured me that these things were 'absolutely normal'. She asked me to calm myself and enjoy the beautiful phase of my impending Motherhood. She prescribed a few medicines to relieve me of those sickening bouts of nausea.

I took the medicines and voila! I was indeed feeling much better. The discomfort was gone. After a long time, I prepared breakfast and relished it in peace. Although I couldn't straightaway resume work but I was feeling much better. I decided to laze around and enjoy being passive all the time.

I passed my days watching movies, listening to music and getting ample rest. I decided to go with the flow and not tax myself too much. I loaded my phone with various maternity apps, which not only helped me understand various things but also helped me keep a track of my baby. It was overwhelming to get to know the developments of the baby every week- the formation of the cute little fingers, the beautiful eyes, ears, the tiny hands, and legs. I was already in love.

I still remember how my husband tolerated my anger and irritability which made me believe:

Pregnancy is a great balance in life. It brings out the worst mood swings in a wife and the best levels of tolerance in a husband.

A note from 'The soon-to-be-father':

After the doctor put all the doubts and confusions to rest, the time had come for both of us to prepare for the arrival of the newest member of our family. However, it was a long way to go yet. Eight months is a long time. In addition, this time would feel even longer for my wife with all the changes her body would go through during her pregnancy. I knew she was going to be unreasonable on occasions and I would have to bear with her. I started voraciously reading anything I could get my hands on to make this time less stressful and more enjoyable for her. I wanted to stay with her as long as I could, talk to her about how wonderful it is all going to be.

One more thing I had to mentally prepare for was not getting enough sleep like I used to. I am a late riser, but this period was changing me since mornings were difficult for my wife. She started complaining about nausea and indigestion. I had read a lot about morning sickness though. The doctor's visit proved to be useful. She gave her a pill that she had to take for the first three months. It gave her a lot of relief. Waking up early in the morning became my habit nevertheless. One at a time, the days were passing and it all felt quite wonderful.

4

Buried Treasure

In spite of my body behaving like crazy, the celebrations were in full swing. However, amidst these happy moments, we received some heart-breaking news. On 18 Feb 2017, at around twelve-thirty in the afternoon, my father-in-law was battling for his life in the Intensive Care Unit of a hospital back home. We were completely shaken by this development. His health was deteriorating by the hour.

I remember, it was a Saturday afternoon. Our lunch was in front of us but neither of us had the appetite for even a single morsel of food. My husband had already booked tickets for the very next day to attend to his ailing father.

'Can I eat it later?' he mumbled.

'I'm not able to eat now, you go ahead please', he added. He gently slid his food aside. Even I didn't want to eat anything but I couldn't let my baby go hungry. Grudgingly, I forced myself to eat a small portion of rice and lentils.

'Let's get ready or else we will be late for the appointment', Subhashish asked me to hurry.

We had a doctor's appointment for a routine check-up. We just went through the grind, our minds and thoughts elsewhere. My husband started his two-wheeler to go to the clinic and I could see the agony and pain on his sullen face. We were on our way when he received a call from his mother. Instinctively, I knew something was wrong. Subhashish could barely mutter a 'Hello' and after a few seconds, the call got disconnected.

He restarted the vehicle, but he couldn't stop the barrage of tears from rolling down.

I could not hold myself back. 'What happened? Who was it?' I demanded.

'Baba is no more'. It was all that he could utter.

His response left me cold. Tears rolled down my cheeks. I was unsure of how to console him at this hour; I felt helpless.

But I had married a strong and brave man. How I wished my father-in-law to be able to see his grandchild. But this was not meant to be. But wherever he would be, my child would always have his blessings.

'Let's go back. We can do this some other day.' I was trying to be helpful and was at a loss of words to console my love.

Although I asked Subhashish to get back home, he would have none of it. He being the ever-responsible father-to-be started towards the clinic. His phone kept ringing. His mother was calling him continuously, distraught. Once inside the clinic, he asked me if I would be comfortable getting the check-up done by myself. I left him alone with his thoughts and emotions.

Subhashish composed himself before calling his mother back.
They both let their emotions flow freely in that hour of grief.

I found him in the parking zone. He was misty-eyed after the call.

'How is mom? Is she all right?', I asked hesitatingly for I knew the answer too.

Can anyone fathom the pain one has to suffer after losing a partner? I shuddered even thinking of it. I couldn't even imagine what my mom-in-law was going through at that point of time.

Once back home, my husband packed his bags and got ready for the tumultuous journey to Assam. Although he was supposed to go the next day, he left that very night. A trip no one can ever prepare oneself for.

By night, I was exhausted. Tired not just physically, but mentally too! I slept with my laptop and phone by my side that night. I wanted to have my husband back beside me even though I knew it was a selfish thought.

Sleep was hard to come by but I tried keeping my eyes closed remembering him in the following way

"I miss you the most at night.

When everything is quiet and the silence reminds me

That I'm not sleeping next to you."

A note from 'The soon-to-be-father':

A month had passed since the first scan and things were going smoothly. I thought I was on top of the situation and well prepared to handle anything that comes up in the next seven months. However, I had never imagined what was coming my way. The demise of my father came as a shock to me. He had been recently discharged from the hospital and with medication, was doing fine. I was expecting him to recover, but his health took a turn for the worse quite abruptly. I had seen him last in the month of January, few days before we got the news that we were pregnant. I had already seen my child playing with his grandfather in my imagination.

Of all the things I was expecting to go through in the months before my child was born, this was the least. My mother and my elder brother were there in Assam, my father died in a hospital in Bhubaneshwar; my uncle was present with my father in his last moments. He was bringing him back to Assam for the cremation.

I wanted to be home as soon as I could. My wife was supportive. She wanted to accompany me but I knew it would be very stressful for her. After many discussions, I decided to head home alone while she stayed back in Bangalore and took care of herself.

5

Half a Month

It was almost two and a half months being pregnant. With the new developments, it wasn't as smooth as I was hoping it to be.

As I was pregnant, I was not supposed to be involved in the mourning process or in the funeral rites. This is done to supposedly safeguard the unborn child. So, I was asked to stay back in Bangalore.

With the demise of my father-in-law, the mental state of everyone in the family was quite disturbed, the atmosphere mournful. And I, back in Bangalore alone, was going through a mix of emotions. My mind too was going through sadness and separation and my heart cried out of melancholy.

Suddenly the phone rang and I rushed albeit carefully to answer. It was my husband.

'Had your breakfast? How is your health?', the concerned voice asked.

'Yeah, I am done with my breakfast and I am alright. I'm missing you', I replied.

I wanted to weep and cry over the phone but didn't. I knew his family needed him now more than ever.

We talked for a few more minutes before hanging up.

I was not in control of my emotions. I felt all of them at once-anger, hunger, and frustration. Not to mention, I was still in my first trimester, the most challenging months of a pregnancy. The mood swings were getting the better of me.

Although I was not physically present at my in-laws' place, my mind was always there. According to our rituals, the mourning family is not supposed to consume regular meals for thirteen days after the funeral. So, even I decided to follow the same. My husband was still there with the family, eating only fruits and Sago. Back here, I started with Sago and bread on the first day. My body rejected it right away and I threw up. Without proper food, I was getting irritated. I somehow passed the day and ate the leftover fruits for dinner.

I tried again the following day. The very thought of eating Sago and fruits made me nauseous. I consulted the family priest who advised me to have rice and boiled potatoes as I should refrain from consuming spices or oil until the thirteenth day after the funeral rites. I love the combination of rice and boiled potato but having the same meal every time killed my appetite for it. By the fifth day, I couldn't take it any longer. My palate was just not up for it.

Earlier, I used to eat every two hours. But now, even though I was hungry, I was too bloated to eat.

Pregnancy makes us crave for some serious pampering, and I was finding it difficult to cope with the situation. The long-distance conversations over the phone were just not enough. Normally, I don't deprive myself of food but the present state of matter was taking away my urge to eat.

I couldn't bring myself to focus on things. My laptop was lying in a corner, books scattered all over my table-my work came to a complete halt. Even at night, I couldn't sleep peacefully as my mind was replete with negative thoughts. As the days passed by, it was becoming increasingly difficult to calm my nerves. My pregnancy hormones wouldn't allow me to go about the daily grind. For some odd reason, a famous quote kept playing on in my mind:

Every minute feels like an hour,
Every hour feels like a day,
Every day feels like forever,
But I will wait forever and a day for you.

Finally, the day arrived when the ritual of breaking the fast was to be observed. It is commemorated by organizing a feast for the priests (Brahmins), relatives and neighbors. This ritual is known as 'Matsamukhi' in our native language. The feast consists of serving fish and other favourite foods of the departed. My mother-in-law made sure that each ritual was followed diligently.

Now, until the priests have had their meal, the others are not served. It was already one-thirty. Since I was so far away from the family, I confirmed over the phone if the priests had eaten. Only then did I serve myself some Chicken Biryani. And it reminded me of my husband. Reluctantly, I ate a few morsels and went to bed.

A Few Days After...

I tried to keep myself busy to keep my thoughts from wandering. I badly needed to see him. I anticipated his arrival every moment. And my happiness knew no bounds when he called me from the airport. He's almost here, I thought. My baby was happy too and let it be known by kicking with his teeny-weeny feet. After long was I experiencing such joy!

It felt as if my little baby was singing:

I'm so glad when daddy comes
home, Glad as I can clap my
hands and Shout for joy.

Then climb upon his knee,
Put my arms around his neck,
Hug him tight like this,
Pat his cheeks then give him
A great big kiss.

A note from 'The soon-to-be-father':

Around two months ago, I had thought that I will always be around my wife in the period of her pregnancy. But as fate would have it, I had to cope with the fact that my father will never be around me again. With a heavy heart, I took the flight for home and after a long day, reached home by evening. In the night, we had the cremation.

The atmosphere at my home town was understandably grim. So many things happened so soon that I almost did not realize what was going on around me, as I was full of grief. Most of my extended family members were present there, all were very supportive. During this period, we needed our friends and family to be together to get over this tragedy.

After cremation, there is a long wait of fourteen days where I was not allowed to eat anything, touch anyone or go outside the house. I only had my brother and my mother for company and we spent the time talking about the past, present and future. After all the rituals got over, I started for Bangalore. My brother was there to take care of my mother. I had to get back to take care of my wife who had been alone in Bangalore for almost a month, while almost three months pregnant.

6

The Homecoming

The whole house was filled with mild fragrances and not because of the potpourris or the room sprays. To welcome my husband after such a long separation, I decided to make the Bengali delicacy- Bengal Carp Curry. The aroma of the Basmati Rice wafted through our home. You might be surprised at this celebration. But after being away for almost a month, Subhashish was finally coming home to me and this definitely called for a celebration.

I am not sure but maybe during pregnancy, you crave for a lot of love, care and attention. No matter how strong and independent you are, during those nine months of your impending motherhood, you want that extra bit of support.

It was almost eleven in the night. I was drowsy with sleep but I tried to stay awake by watching a movie. The minutes were getting longer. Finally, the door-bell rang. I made a dash towards the door. The moment was magical. Seeing him after so long brought tears of happiness and they flowed unchecked. I felt as if I was meeting him after years.

'How are you? How have you been?'

'You are asking me as if we are meeting after ages', he giggled.

'That's why I always ask you not to fight with me, you never know when I will be gone', he said with a wink.

I knew he was fooling me emotionally but my pregnancy hormones spare no one.

After Subhashish freshened up, I called him for dinner. A meal that I had so lovingly prepared and was dying to share it with him! The first morsel satiated me in a way a beggar would be satiated when served a 'royal' meal. I guess it is the company that matters. Sharing one of our favourite meals left us both contented and happy.

After ages, I could finally sleep peacefully. My love was back in my arms and I couldn't ask for more. The bedtime discussions, jokes, and our sit-coms were on!

A note from 'The soon-to-be-father':

It was a long time since I had seen my wife. Although she was very supportive and always said things are very normal whenever we talked over the phone, I knew it was difficult for her to manage everything alone. The trauma of losing my father had not passed completely from my mind. But there was this realization that he is in a better place and will be showering blessings on us from there as I become a father myself.

The journey was long and tiring. It's a four-hour drive from my hometown to the airport and then the flight itself was with a four-hour layover at Kolkata. I started in the morning and by the time I reached home in Bangalore, it was late in the evening. I knew Banani would definitely cook for me, but I didn't imagine she would prepare such a sumptuous meal. And she herself hadn't eaten dinner. Although the gesture was very loving, I had to be a little upset because she should have been taking her meals on time. Anyway, after we had our dinner together, we finally retired to bed.

7

Negative Feelings

I was on the verge of completing my first trimester and was about to enter the next phase. I regained my energy, started feeling more active than the previous months, left the morning sickness far behind and experienced no more prolonged sleep and lethargy. The pleasure of having breakfast together with my husband was back.

Those days, my kickass mornings used to start by seven. Listening to Joel Osteen lifted my spirits up and I would be all set to start my day with new zeal. One full glass of water and a big bowl of muesli with milk helped build my immunity and satisfy my hunger.

The weekends weren't much different but the breakfast menu certainly did change. I preferred savoring 'Dosa' with piping hot 'Sambar' and coconut chutney. And at other times, my tongue craved for fluffy hot 'Pooris' with potato sabji.

'Paratha and Chicken Curry', I muttered to myself almost like a zombie. My mind was having a monologue with my stomach. One evening while waiting for my husband, I had a strong urge to have home-made parathas and chicken curry. I was in an impossible situation as I was feeling too lazy to cook.

I called my husband who was on his way home and let him know about my craving.

'Who will cook chicken now? Should I get it from a restaurant?' he asked in a tensed voice.

'I want my mom's chicken curry', I cried in an irritating voice and disconnected the call. Pregnancy hormones, you see. They make an appearance when you least expect them.

Pregnancy is when you are officially allowed to swear and scream at your husband and blame it all on hormones.

My chicken curry was on its way and I somehow managed to prepare those parathas. That night, I had almost two and a half parathas to satisfy myself. I grabbed my plate like a hungry dog and those big parathas with the chicken curry made way to my stomach within seconds. I cannot describe in words the effect of that meal.

But then suddenly something happened! I was unable to move. Neither could I breathe properly nor walk after that heavy dinner. My upper abdomen became as rigid and strong as JK tyres. I tried lying down on the bed and rest but I simply couldn't. The first thought that ran through my mind was, 'Am I having a heart attack?' My chest had been congested for almost an hour by then. Every possible turbulent feeling was going through my mind.

My husband was terrified and didn't have a clue as to what was happening that night. He offered me some water and suggested that we visit the nearest hospital. The idea of visiting the hospital scared me and I broke into a cold sweat. Was it something serious? I had no idea.

'Eat small quantities and feed yourself every two hours' the doctor advised. Ah! Those golden words of my gynaecologist were music to my ears. I had finally found the clue to my queasy situation.

But it was better said than done. The hunger pangs were back with gusto, but the acidity just wouldn't go away.

'I have to be a little cautious about what and when I am popping into my mouth', I bit my lower lip and gave it a deep thought. I decided to escape my husband's scolding and hence did not reveal the reason the same day. I passed a gentle smile and decided to close my eyes and drift away into sleep.

Next morning, I woke up healthy and happy. The sunlight was streaming through the white curtains welcoming a bright new day.

As I was back to my normal routine, I believed my laptop was a lot happier than I was, to get back to work as it lay unused for many days. It was covered with a thin sheath of dust which I cleaned lovingly with a plain muslin cloth before hitting the keys. I spent time working, reading books, cooking and watching some Hindu Mythological series. Long story short, I was happy with this phase of transition.

Along with the beautiful changes, came along a few shortcomings. My lips were getting dry just like the old withered leaves of autumn. Initially, I thought my body was getting dehydrated but fortunately, that was not the case. My doctor suggested drinking plenty of fluids and juices, however, it didn't work either. Tired of trying everything, I decided to do some intensive research of my own.

The Internet proved to be my friend as I voraciously read most of the reputed articles on pregnancy. I found the answer to my problem- a tube of lip balm. And whoa! it worked. Much ado but nothing, I grinned at myself.

However, on the other hand, my mind was a tangled mess with certain peculiar things- the intermittent stress, the jealousy, the not-so-good feeling about labour, failure, frustration- all negative feelings just hovered over me throughout the day. I was clueless and confused about those bizarre thoughts of mine.

I had to calm myself down as the thoughts of the mother affect the baby too! The baby feels down when the mother is unhappy and irritated. If you are lazy in your pregnancy, your baby turns out to be lethargic. This is not my theory alone but with Google vouching for it too! It became quite important to be surrounded by pleasant ways of living. It can be watching a comic series or reading good books, the choice is yours. To have a happy pregnancy, you have to keep yourself happy.

When I spoke to my husband about my negative feelings, he assured me that every thing's going to be fine. He asked me to watch a few positive videos which might help me get rid of the junk in my head.

'Cut off all the connections that give you negative vibes', he advised.

I felt my brain would freeze whenever there's a dominant fear of failure, be it in starting my own venture or the temptation to buy a new house or a luxurious car like my friends. I was never so negative about my strengths and potential. All my life I have never had the slightest attraction towards materialistic things. I was rather fascinated with the idea of traveling around the globe.

What was wrong with me? I felt like a rudderless ship in the middle of the Pacific ocean. At times, I suspected someone of performing black magic on me and what not! Was it really me after all? The answer was-'Yes, it was me, high on HCG.'

A note from 'The soon-to-be-father':

It was that time when getting dozens of calls in a day from my wife while I was at office was becoming the new normal. Most of the calls were just rants about random things. I would always try to calm her down while she went on and on about something.

Up until the time when you can start feeling the baby move, it's not really real for you. What is going on in there? I have read a lot about hormonal changes in a pregnant woman, but it was still baffling for me to see her change so often so soon. It’s like I am sharing space with three-four different women in one body.

I would try to get her the things she craved for. But that was tricky as the cravings would change by the time I got her favourite things. Then she would crave for something else. I could not show irritation on my face because that would have made her mad and she'd spend the next two hours letting me know how I had made her feel.

Having a pregnant wife at home will always make your office work take the lower priority. It is difficult to manage. I had made a firm rule of not taking any office work back home. Whenever I was at home, my time was only for my wife and my future child.

This is the time when a lot of emphasis is given on being strong mentally.

8

Cold War

Grrrrrrrrrrrr! Grrrrrrrrrr! I was extremely embarrassed about continuously making those sounds but I couldn't help it. I could feel the cab driver getting irritated with the continuous nose-blowing. My nose was stuffed but I was battle ready with my pack of tissues. My husband asked me to go easy on the blowing as I might get a headache. My nose was filled with mucus, making it difficult to sit comfortably even for a few seconds. I was caught up in this war between my immune system and the unknown virus. For the last two weeks, it was getting crazier by the day.

The following Sunday, we were headed towards Hotel Marriott for a Prenatal workshop organized by Cloud Nine Hospitals and it took us almost an hour to reach there. The cab was moving at a snail's pace due to the crazy traffic in the city. I was getting agitated because I was running a temperature, my nose was blocked and the continuous honking of the vehicles was getting on my nerves. In spite of the AC in the cab, I was hot. I was jittery.

Haichoo! Haichoo! my nose was continuously emitting tiny infectious droplets and the clogged mucous was making my breathing uncomfortable.

'How long will it take for us to reach?' I was getting restless.

'Another 10 minutes madam', the driver answered.

'Oh yes. Even Google says the same.'

After a few minutes, we finally reached our destination. We walked towards the conference room and were politely greeted by the executives of Cloud Nine. It was such a delightful scene with all those women carrying their babies and being accompanied by their husbands.

Flowing Maxi dresses, knee-length summer dresses, bright coloured Anarkalis and what not? Someone rightly said, *'Every day is a fashion show, and the world is your runway'.*

The cold-shouldered dress of my neighbour was particularly appealing. She was flaunting her baby bump and looked marvellous! I was checking out almost everyone's outfit in that big room and I felt a little under dressed for the occasion in those simple black jeggings and a light pink top. All those mums-to-be were nothing short of style icons and I made a mental note to go shopping at the first chance.

'When are you taking me shopping?', I asked my husband who was deeply engrossed in the manual provided by the centre. The unexpected question almost surprised him.

'Will go for sure but not today', he replied and resumed what he was involved in.

I was making a mental list of things to buy-preparing myself to look gorgeous in this wonderful state of Motherhood.

Within no time, the speaker took charge of the dais and started the session. She took us through the dietary guidelines for pregnancy and whoa! I gathered some very nice information. Talking about food, my hormones started the happy dance to signal that I was hungry. We were served a hot and healthy breakfast and finally, both my tummy and my tiny baby inside were satisfied.

We were back in the conference room to attend the rest of the session. Uff! My nose started troubling me again. I had cleaned my nose before entering the room but to my surprise, it started irritating me again. I can't blow my nose here, in this room full of people, I thought to myself. I was itching to blow my nose and without second thoughts, I took out a tissue and went for it with full gusto.

I didn't know about the rest but my neighbour gave me a disgusted look. Although she didn't say anything, her expression asked me to keep the virus to myself. I couldn't do anything but look away.

The speakers spoke a lot about stem cell banking, nutrition, etc. but the best part was the pre-natal exercise session. The practitioner gave demonstrations and asked us to do the same with our respective husbands. With all that stretching, I was relaxed and felt good. Like everyone else in the room, even we both enjoyed the session. After some time, we all proceeded for lunch.

I didn't have the courage to attend the next session not because I was not well or the sessions were boring, but because the next session was called 'Labour' and I didn't have the guts to sit through it. I didn't want to know what actually happens in the labour room. I had 'googled' about labour and whatever I had learned had left me nauseated and nervous. I didn't want to stress myself and hence, decided to skip.

Back home I took some rest, applied some vaporizer followed by steam. My eyes were tired, my puffy nose as red as a tomato. I somehow managed to sleep that night hoping to get well soon.

A note from 'The soon-to-be-father':

Cloud Nine is one of the most trusted speciality hospitals for pregnancy and child-care. From the very first day, we have always consulted the same doctor in the same hospital. I preferred it over any multi-speciality hospital. I had made my mind that we would have our baby delivered at Cloud Nine. So I had booked a package with them at the outset which included pre-delivery check-ups, delivery, post-delivery care and more.

As a part of that, we were entitled to a pre-natal workshop. These workshops are really useful in getting rid of most of the misconceptions you might have about pregnancy and also most of the myths that are sufficiently widespread. A misconception that I had was that a woman just needs to rest and stay idle when she is pregnant. That myth was busted in the workshop. Even if you are pregnant, you need proper exercise to stay healthy, which would also help the baby. The presentation on the workout was good and informative.

I liked the part where the nutrition expert talked about all the food you can have and things to avoid during pregnancy. Overall, it was a good session to attend. It was a full day event and after the long day, we could finally go home where Banani's running nose got some rest.

9

The Chase Begins

Baby I don't need dollar bills to have fun tonight (I love cheap thrills)
Baby I don't need dollar bills to have fun tonight (I love cheap thrills)
But I don't need no money
As long as I can feel the beat
I don't need no money
As long as I keep dancing

The music was on; I started tapping my foot, and grooving slowly in my kitchen. I was surrounded by veggies, holding a shining stainless steel knife and a chopping board- all set to prepare a delicious lunch for myself and my cherub inside.

Cooking de-stresses me, it's an art for me and pregnancy gave me new goals to cook- healthy drinks, easy one-pot meals, effortless mini snacks to relish and delicious multi-cuisines with gusto. As much as I love devouring good food, I immensely enjoy cooking too. I believe *'Cooking is at once a child's play and an adult's joy. And cooking done with care is an act of love.'*

In the midst of chopping a bunch of coriander leaves to garnish the chicken curry, I felt a few gas bubbles pop inside my stomach.

'What's that?' I was a little surprised. I ignored it at first assuming it to be gas or acidity that had troubled me quite so often.

After some time, the gas bubbles crawled to another part of my tummy. The bubbles stopped and then started again. I stood quietly for some time, pressing my right palm on my belly only for it to happen again and then the sensation disappeared. Now I was convinced that I was facing some stomach issues. I witnessed a pattern. Whenever I did something with great concentration, the bubbles came back popping. I didn't pay much attention to them and continued watching my favourite shows. I was unsure of the gesticulation.

It was that time of my pregnancy when I had to visit the hospital for my antenatal scan, blood sugar test, and vaccination. Before starting for the hospital, I gulped the glucose solution given to me the previous day, to be consumed two hours prior to the blood test. Once I reached, the nurse called me in for the vaccination and I was nervous as usual. Thankfully, the prick of the needle wasn't too painful and the process didn't take much time.

'Keep your muscles relaxed, don't stiffen yourself', the nurse commanded drawing the drug into the syringe.

The nurse injected the needle and pushed the piston delivering the drug into my broad arms.

'Are you okay?' Subhashish looked worried.

And I replied with my shaky voice, 'Yes, I'm fine.'

Once we were done with the vitals and vaccination, both of us were ready for the most exciting part of our visit - the scan, where we would get to meet our baby. Excited and elated, we both entered the room. I lay down on the bed next to the big computer screen and Subhashish adjusted himself in a corner seat to get a clear picture of the baby. The doctor was already ready with the transducer covered in gel. Just a few more minutes and we can finally meet our baby, I thought excitedly. However, to my disappointment, our baby was not ready to show up his face that day. He hid his face with his tiny little hands. The little hands were up near his ears fencing his face. Our expectant eyes were eagerly waiting.

'Why isn't the baby showing his face?' I was disheartened.

'Let me try once again', the doctor said patiently.

But it was just not happening.

The doctor was kind enough to ask us to visit again after half an hour. We both decided to finish our lunch and returned within the stipulated time. My heart sank, feeling sad with disappointment. Why not? After a long couple of weeks, I desperately wanted to see our baby. Regular scanning is not advised and we would have to wait until the appropriate time comes for the ultrasound.

Back in the hospital, I was praying fervently to God to let me have a look at my baby's face at least once.

The would-be-father gave me a quick glance and we both exchanged assuring smiles before entering the room. Deep inside our hearts, we both knew that we were praying hard!

Again, I lay on the bed and the doctor rolled the scanning device over my belly. We could see the baby with the face still hidden. I felt as if the baby was playing hide and seek with us. This time, the doctor played a trick. She asked me to cough a bit. I coughed very gently and hurray! My baby showed its face as if he could sense my voice. It was such a wonderful thing to happen.

My husband and I cheered with joy. It was a beautiful moment for us.

As scheduled, we had to visit our gynaecologist the following day with all our medical test reports. This time she checked for the baby's heartbeats with an instrument that sounded more like a military walkie-talkie when placed on my belly and yes, I could hear the heart beating!

Though the medical test results were normal, I was curious to know about the gas bubbles whose origin was still unknown.

'I can feel some air bubbles popping inside my stomach, is it gas?' I was really curious to know.

'No, those are the movements of your little one', she confirmed. Nearing twenty weeks, you start feeling the movements a bit, she added further.

There were goosebumps all over my body. A chill went down my spine. My eyes teary, with joy, of course, and my heart beating with double its speed. I so wished to rush to a room and lock myself up just to let that moment sink in. But I somehow controlled my emotions. That moment cannot be described in words. A life inside me was forming gradually; it was moving, responding and who knows my baby must have already started playing within its tiny area!

There is no better feeling than to be able to feel those movements. A new phase had started in the journey of motherhood where I was being able to communicate with my baby. I would always wait for the movements and whenever they happened, I would gently rub my belly as if to say, 'Mom is right here with you'. I passed my days chasing those movements and would be disheartened when I couldn't feel them.

Seeing my gloomy face, my husband would cheer me up saying, 'Our baby is sleeping now. It sleeps for almost twenty hours, you know.'

At night we both would play with the baby. The would-be father would narrate bed-time stories, shower me and my baby with goodnight kisses and we would all doze off together. I waited for the movements as eagerly and restlessly as I would have waited as for any expected guests to ring the doorbell.

There is no better feeling than feeling my baby move around in my womb, I must say!

I read these beautiful lines somewhere which stayed on in my mind:

I Am Not Alone

Running errands and talking on the phone,

I am pleasantly reminded that I am not alone.
Little tiny hands a precious rounded knee
Pushing and twisting that no one can see.
Oh sweet child kicking up your heels,
It is our sweet little secret that only I can feel.
I look forward to your birth,

When I can kiss your skin,
But for now, I will just smile,
As I feel you play within.

A note from 'The soon-to-be-father':

I remembered the last time we went for an ultrasound scan. We could hear a heartbeat and was able to see a black dot. It did give goose bumps at that time, but it did not look anything like a baby. Now, after so many months, I hoped to get a different result.

We have been visiting the doctor quite regularly. We have been doing everything that she advised. I wanted to find out what is happening with the little one in there. So, when the doctor prescribed an ultrasound, I was excited.

So we reached the hospital on time on the day of the scan. However, the little guy was in no mood to show up so easily. It took us multiple attempts and lot of efforts to get a good view but it was satisfying in the end. We were able to see the baby move. We were able to see the limbs and the face. It was overwhelming. I just could not wait for the next few weeks to pass so that I could hold my baby in my arms.

10

Babymoon

It was a usual morning, I was alone at home working on my next article. Keeping my laptop aside I found myself drawn towards the balcony. The soothing breeze kissed my cheeks and to my joy, it started drizzling. The gentle drops of rain gave me a feeling of freshness, contentment, and joy. It ushered in a sense of sheer happiness after the hot and humid summer. The glass windows sparkled with thick crystal-like raindrops.

The wind started blowing hard, sweeping the dust off the road. The trees were bending and dancing to the rhythm of the flowing wind. The dark clouds rumbled in the distant sky. Forks of lightning were electrifying the sky, the birds hurried to their nests and the labourers from the nearby construction site managed to hide under the half-constructed shade.

I stood there doing nothing but gazing at the way the slight drizzle gave way to a heavy downpour. The clattering sound of the raindrops was music to my ears. Everyone and everything got drenched in this downpour- the lake at the front, the canopy of the coconut trees and the tall buildings. Slowly, the vision was getting blurred due to the extensive force of the thunderstorm.

As long as I was standing there, I almost forgot about my little one inside until he made me realize his existence with his tiny movements. The right side of my stomach shook a bit which broke my concentration. The baby too started enjoying the downpour, I felt.

I came inside after some time and continued to complete the half-written piece on 'Monsoon Diaries'.

My husband and I were both busy with our own lives during the day but used to relax together in the evenings. I wanted more time with him and our baby, which I was unable to have. In fact, the more time I had, the more I craved. I became a greedy wife - greedy for peace of mind, time and love.

The thought of making my venture, which I had started almost three years back, a significant one didn't allow me to sleep. My thoughts intersected with each other and occupied my mind-business, pregnancy, excellence, motherhood, and labour.
I wanted to shut out all my thoughts and escape.

It was almost six months since I had last put on my travelling shoes. I considered myself almost a vagabond, it was nearly impossible for me to lead a life without travelling for months but this time the reason was good enough to resist my travel temptations. It was hard to make up my mind, though!

But finally one fine day, we three- I, my husband and our baby-were all set to escape to somewhere far from the hustle and bustle of the city, but only after my doctor's approval.

That Saturday morning around six-thirty, we started our journey to the Western Ghats, the Malnad region of Karnataka. Our destination was the Golden Woods Resort, Sakleshpur. Never in my life had I ever spent any vacation at a resort- doing almost nothing. I always had a notion that visiting a place, lazing around, without any adventure or exploration can't be a vacation. This was until I spent those two days in Sakleshpur.

We hired a bigger vehicle for the trip in order to comfort my body, especially my back, and the baby. With ample leg-room, I could stretch my legs comfortably. I carried a large handbag and my camera without which I couldn't survive. My husband was carrying a medium-sized travel bag. We didn't want to overburden ourselves.

As I was adjusting myself next to the left window, Suhashish asked me if I was comfortable. Yes, I was.

The weather of that early summer morning was refreshing. The drive on the highway recharged my cells as I had come out of my home after a really long time. I rolled down my window and was enjoying the endless roads, the fellow travellers and the mesmerizing nature around us. After a drive of almost an hour and a half, my stomach growled with hunger.

'I think the baby has woken up. It's moving and demanding some breakfast,' I grinned at my husband.

But my husband knew me well.

'Oh yes! Only the baby must be hungry and not you, right?' he asked, teasingly.

We stopped at a roadside hotel where many families and travellers flocked. Few were sitting inside and sipping their morning tea and filling their stomach with hot, white, puffy round idlis. We chose our table and grabbed our seat before anyone else could. We invited our chauffeur to join us which he politely declined. But upon my request, he finally came and took a seat at our table. He felt a little awkward in our company.

The aroma of pure ghee coming from the kitchen wafted through my nostrils. I couldn't wait any longer and asked my husband to place the order immediately.

'Three Masala Dosa, two tea, and a bottle of mineral water please,' my husband placed the order.

The waiter was in his 40s, a medium-sized dark man with round bulging eyes like those of a frog. He repeated and confirmed our order and left the table.

After a wait of almost 10 minutes, arrived the 'Dosa'- the big, light brown coloured folded pancake made with rice batter. It was hollow from both the sides so that one could peep from either side. It was accompanied by two small bowls- one with coconut chutney and the other with hot, tangy, sweet sambhar. The waiter was quick and active. The Dosa was soft and the chutney and sambar were just perfect for the breakfast. What a nice start to the day!

'Do you need anything else?' Subhashish asked as he knew of my growing appetite.

I shook my head refusing more food.

Our chauffeur was ready, his hands were on the steering wheel while my husband and I made ourselves comfortable at the back. We drove for almost three hours. I slept, gazed out the window, hummed my favourite tunes and slept on and off. Witnessing a baffling bazaar - the confusion in the streets, the shopkeepers, the sudden blowing of horns of the buses, made me realize that we had entered the city, Sakleshpur. The Google map directed us to drive for another 4 km to reach the homestay. To our surprise, the road was under construction. The caretakers of the homestay guided us on the phone and we followed a different route.

The other road was bumpy, covered with both small gravel and big stones with sharp edges. There were muddy potholes, which lay undetected to the outsider. I was nervous about the jerks. I held my bump tightly, praying fervently. My husband was getting irritated and anxious about the constant jolts and jerks of the vehicle.

'I'm getting scared because of madam's condition', our driver said pensively.

He was driving gently and smoothly.

'You are doing well, nothing will happen. Don't worry.' I assured him.

He was steering the wheel with utmost care. In spite of myself being at the edge of fear, I gave a quick glance to my husband and assured him of the same.

I preferred not showing any signs of nervousness and fear on my face even though I was.

After many jolts and bolts on our way, the vehicle finally took a silent halt. We took off our minimal luggage and I heaved a sigh of relief after that bumpy ride. The ride would have been fun but with them little one in my womb, it turned out to be a bit scary and risky too. After all, there's a living being inside, growing gradually! Without much ado, we then headed towards the homestay. The property had four gorgeous rooms built on different and unique themes. We were given 'The Brick Cottage', which was supposedly the most 'romantic' one, the one I had been eyeing for so long.

It was around twelve-thirty by my watch when we entered the room. We took a quick shower to skim off the weariness of the journey. The host welcomed us and asked us to join her for a delicious lunch. The timing was perfect as my baby had started showing signs of hunger. We were escorted towards a nearby stream where perfect seating arrangements had been made and the food was ready to be served. Rice, Chappatis, Fish Curry, Chicken Masala, Vegetable Curry-everything was served one after another.

'Everything here is grown organically. Except for the meat which we buy from the nearby market, we grow everything here. The area is plastic-free and even our electricity is hydro-generated,' the host informed us proudly. I was happy to visit such a nice place during my babymoon. Even the baby was gaining some knowledge, I grinned to myself.

It was a hearty lunch, I must say.

'Let me take you guys around the estate,' the host offered.

But both my husband and the owner were apprehensive and doubted whether I would be able to walk.

'I'll be fine. Just be with me,' I assured my husband.

It was a very small trek along the stream which gave way to a small lake and a meadow. The sight was beautiful and serene, my heart could barely leave the place. We listened patiently to the host mentioning her future plans regarding the property. After a while we trekked down; I, holding the hands of my husband and at times, the hosts'.

The short trek was followed by a quick ride around the estate. I sat in the front seat to avoid the jerking. The host took charge of the driver's seat and my husband sat at the back. Jeep rides are fun in the hills but could be risky for a pregnant lady. I was lucky to have such an understanding host who took care of me like an elder sister. But I would not advise such a drive for an expectant mom.

'These are Arabica and the smaller leaves are those of the Robusta,' the host mentioned while taking us around the estate.

After parking the jeep on the side of the road we descended from the vehicle. We then followed her towards the coffee plantation area. Both sides of the road were covered with lush green vegetation and she took us for a leisurely walk around the estate informing and educating us about everything regarding the coffee plantation.

'We also grow other plants like cardamom, cloves, peppercorns, coconut, betel nuts which help in conserving the vegetation. They aid our coffee plants and also help in preserving the natural habitat of the wild animals,' the host informed helpfully. This is an elephant prone area, she added.

She took us to their factory, their lab and we ended our tour with a cup of hot, aromatic and freshly brewed coffee. We visited the other home-stays in the estate and picked one for my next stay after my little one arrives.

After the knowledge and experience sharing, she dropped us back at our little abode for that day. I was a bit tired but was feeling relaxed- no laptop, no mobile, no T.V- nothing. I could have hardly imagined myself like this before. Never did I think that I would be so happy without these inanimate and materialistic things. I had found a new me!

Since we gained a lot of knowledge that day, we hoped that our baby learned something new too.

We both went off to bed for a short nap.

It was evening and the clouds started grumbling. The sky turned dark grey and I found both of us still slumped on the bed. I felt nearly unconscious and was trying to gather my scattered thoughts.

'Sir, tea, sir', one of the caretakers knocked at our door. My husband slid from the bed and marched towards the door.

'Sir, you want tea? We will also serve pakodas', the voice on the other side of the door informed my husband.

'Yes, two cups of tea, please.' The moment I heard the word 'pakodas' I jumped out of my slumber, became active and sat straight with my back to the wall.

'After such a long time I am going to have pakodas,' I excitedly told my husband.

'Yes. You can have it but eat carefully or else you will complain of severe gastric pain later.' How can anyone have any idea about my pakoda craving!

I remember that horrible night when I had to go through a terrible gastric pain attack. When the oily, deep fried golden pakodas arrived, my mouth wouldn't stop watering and within no time I finished almost four big pieces of those. I failed to resist the temptation. Ah! How do I describe that moment? It was just perfect for a leisurely vacation- the rains had started, the whole forest was drenched, the room was getting darker, the temperature came down, a soothing breeze flowed and we both sat together sipping the hot masala tea paired with pakodas, gazing at the rains pouring down cats and dogs. With every single bite, my soul was delighted.

We spoke, chatted, discussed infinitely after so long. There was no fear of our talks getting disrupted by any pesky phone calls or any assignment submissions. Overall, I fell in love with the place and with my man all over again!

As soon as the rains stopped, the campfire was all set to be lit. The daylight ceased and night pulled over. The weather became calm and cool. The earthy smell was fresh and exhilarating. The mango trees stood proudly, loaded with juicy mangoes. Its leaves held thick rain droplets. The jackfruit trees surrounding the property were no competition. It was only the chirping of crickets that one could hear. The silence of the dense forest engulfed us. There were a couple of other guests on the property. We all gathered around the campfire.

A delicious meal was served at dinner time- pork curry and coconut cakes, something that I was waiting for. There were other dishes too but I picked my favorites to satiate my hunger and temptation.

Afterwards, we took a leisurely walk, accompanied by jokes, fun and mischief.

'Do you remember our school days when you used to bring chocolates for me?' I started the conversation reminiscing about the many childhood memories of us together.

'I wish we could go back in time', he replied holding my hands in his.

During our school days we never realized that we were making memories, we just knew we were having fun just like the other lovebirds.

That night we spoke about our flirty messages, romantic dates, good-night calls, talking about our destiny, those priceless moments, the sweet memories, the cute cuddles, life sans worries, sudden short-lived break-ups and planning for our future.

We talked, listened, shared and talked again.

We both walked towards our cottage for a good night's sleep. I took my iron tablets like every day.

The would-be father read stories to our little one, the one who might be listening curiously to each and every word inside.

Once upon a time, there was a girl called Radha. Her lovely, old grandma was poor and was feeling unwell. Radha decided to visit her and she took a basket of flowers to make her feel better...

The story continued.

I fell asleep within no time, delving deep into my dreams- into the world of fantasy, hallucinations and stupor.

A note from 'The soon-to-be-father':

What do you need most when you've been pregnant for more than five months? I have been juggling my work and personal life for quite some time. It had become mechanical. Most of the day, I was at work and spent the late evenings and night at home. Whenever I was at home, we talked about the pregnancy, the baby and how it was going to change our lives. After that, I read stories to the baby and then, we went to sleep.

The vacation was something that we were both looking forward to. I was a little sceptical as well as the journey was long and I was not sure how tiring the journey was going to be. I was not wrong as the roads leading up to the resort were indeed very bad. Thankfully, our driver understood the situation. He drove very carefully and when we reached the destination, we were pleasantly surprised at how beautiful the place was. It was a much needed break from our routine life and we enjoyed every moment of it. It was not a long vacation, but two days of stress busting was all I could afford at that stage.

11

Getting Back Home

Next morning at around six-thirty, I opened my eyes with difficulty but loved the way I was proving to be a sloth in bed, thinking about nothing. I could only admire the musical heavy pouring outside. It reminded me of the clattering sound the rains made on the tin roof at my parents' place. It was my love affair with the rains, which somehow turned sour once I shifted to Bangalore. I think I had forgotten to observe, feel, write and make memories. Even today, in its absence, I could feel those loud clattering sounds on my roof. I closed my eyes which took me back to my school days. Nostalgia engulfed me.

'Majoni, dorja aaru khirki bondho kora.' (In Assamese, it means- Close the doors and windows, dear daughter), my mom used to scream from the other room. We could hardly hear each other because of the incessant rain. When it rained, the big teak trees in front of our house used to sway violently in the wind. Although I sometimes felt scared, I loved the way the rain used to augment. Diligently, I used to close all the doors and windows except the one in front of my study table. I always kept it open until the raindrops came howling into my room.

The road bore the brunt of the heavy downpour, creating ripples in the nearby canals. Neighbours would come out of their house to gather the clothes from the clothesline. Half-naked toddlers hurried to their homes, covering their heads with big colocasia leaves. The neighbourhood kids loved floating paper boats in the puddles.

My dad is an experimental cook and seldom went wrong with his experiments. He has special dishes for each and every season and occasion. So then how could the monsoons be left out? My dad's Masala Puffed Rice was a big hit during most of the lazy monsoon evenings- puffed rice, chopped raw onions, chopped green chillies, chopped coriander leaves, Chanachur (a type of mixed lentils and peanuts). After a dash of lemon juice and a quick mix, the delicious snack was ready. I, my brother and my parents, we all used to relish the snack while enjoying the rains outside. I would go back to my study table only to view the outside through my window as I loved to observe and make memories.

'Honey, get up! It's eight already. It's time to move or else we will be late.'

Suddenly, my thoughts were interrupted and I came back to reality.

'Get up! Let's freshen up and march towards the breakfast table', Subhashish smirked.

Opening my eyes with much difficulty, I peeped outside from the sides of the curtain. The rain had stopped. The birds came out of their nests, the sky was clear but still there was no sign of a bright sunshine. I was in love with the weather that I used to hate earlier. It was the sign of a typically gloomy day in Bangalore. Ah! I got it, this was a new me, I suppose.

My little cherub inside started his tiny movements signalling his hunger as his mom too needed some breakfast. I softly patted on my stomach as if replying to his messages and assuring him of a delicious breakfast soon. To my surprise, nowadays, the baby responds to my gestures by stopping his fast movements and waits for his food. If it got a little late, he would knock against the womb as if to remind me of something I had forgotten.

We got ready, packed our bags and headed towards the dining area. The morning couldn't have been better with the puffy hot pooris and potato curry, bread and omelette and Poha (flattened rice pulao). After almost an hour, we bade everyone goodbye until the next time and set out on another journey.

After leaving that place, we headed towards Belur and Haleibeidu which was almost 50kms from Saklcshpur. This was not included in our plan but I so wanted to extend my vacation that I didn't want to go back home so early. My partner understood and nodded his head in approval. The places were famous because of their historical importance. The temples, their architecture, the small town- it had a certain character to it and was a nice experience. For me, I wanted to extend the journey as much as I could, especially the drive on the endless roads with my partner by my side. What more could I ask for, knowing very well that after returning to the city, the monotonous, busy life was going to replace the peace, relaxation and the simplicity of this life.

We took a midway to grab some lunch at a local restaurant. The food didn't disappoint and after filling our tummies, we started to traverse the rest of the journey. The roads were broad, clean and green along the sides. The chauffeur was driving the vehicle consciously and carefully, keeping in mind my little one and me, of course.

As we were nearing the completion of our trip, we witnessed the traffic which claimed that we had entered the city. The smooth drive was replaced by a continuously interrupted one. There was barely any greenery outside. All I could see were frustrating faces saddled on to their respective vehicles. We were all headed in the same direction.

We finally reached our home after much effort. We were tired and I hardly had the energy to cook, so we ordered dinner from outside. The much-needed vacation was not only a babymoon for me but it turned out to be instrumental in finding the real me, the one which I had lost somewhere in the innocence of Assam and its dense jungles years ago.

A vacation can be purely a leisurely one rather than an adventurous one. And now I was in love with leisure which I had somehow forgotten to enjoy. This trip reminded me- *'All happiness lies in a leisurely breakfast.'*

The unborn baby had started teaching me everything! If I wouldn't have conceived I wouldn't have demanded a much-needed travel break nor could I have understood and enjoyed the fun of leisure travel. I have always loved speed but at that point, I realized that there is more to life than speeding ahead.

The much-needed sleep was pulling me towards it but I was in my own whimsical world- trying to observe, feel, write and make memories.

A note from 'The soon-to-be-father':

The worst thing about any vacation is that it has to end. After a very relaxing stay at Sakhleshpur, we were going back to Bangalore. I knew well that this could be last time we were travelling outside the city before the big day. The delivery was still a few months away. We had a lot of things in mind that needed to be done before that. Most of our time together was spent discussing the routine doctor visits, the growth of the baby and stuff like what to eat and what not. This short break from our routine life had given us an opportunity to just forget everything and relax. Too bad it was getting over.

12

It's Time to Educate Myself

'*See no evil, hear no evil and do no evil'*, these words of my mom hummed like mantras in my ears. Whenever she phoned or visited during my pregnancy, the only thing she insisted on was to shut out all the negative energies. She asked me to read good books but not restrict myself to the religious ones. She asked me to listen to melodious music and also advised me to refrain from indulging in gossips and arguments.

'The baby is attached to you and would be affected by whatever you think, speak and indulge yourself in', my mom used to warn me.

Even though it's not scientifically proven but there are theories that say that unborn babies may retain some information or even the taste of certain foods after their birth, with the fear of getting my baby affected by the so-called negative energies, I tried my best not to get involved in any sort of nuisance. But you attract the energies that you give off!

I had changed. Even the most routine conversations would infuriate me. Only a few jokes could make me laugh. It was as if the humorous side of me was gone. Suddenly I had gone from being a neutral person to being very judgmental and my anger wouldn't leave me. These pregnancy hormones were making me crazy!

Since an idle brain is the devil's workshop, it became quite important to calm my mind and keep it occupied. To caress the ripples in my mind, I thought of educating myself on my impending motherhood. I didn't want my motherhood to become an excuse for hunger, irritation or sleeplessness but I wanted to make it a strong reason to educate myself and to be a better person than the day before. Needless to say, this tiny little creature inside had made me discover many different facets of life and most importantly, about myself which I was not aware of until then.

To educate your baby, you need to educate yourself first and as someone rightly said, 'Children learn more from what you are than what you teach.' What better way to enjoy pregnancy than to learn and unlearn stuff?

I started to fill in the gaps with whatever I had missed doing all these years. It could be watching an animated movie, reading a famous book or learning to play a new indoor game. I was making myself aware so that my newborn baby need not depend on gadgets or crave for any external help. Initially, I wanted my baby to get to know things from its own home and surroundings, be it a formal education or any form of skill-set. Like every mom, I would like to be the best teacher for my child and to do so it became quite important to educate myself in the right way.

Family problems, work pressure and an increased restlessness due to growing responsibilities can result in a lot of negativity. I was no different. Even I had to deal with them which sometimes became tough to handle. But we strong women somehow always manage to come out of the crap!

The first thing I tried to inculcate in myself was to make myself calm, irrespective of the situation. Trust me, it wasn't as easy as it sounds. Being quite impulsive by nature, I seldom used to give a second thought before doing or saying anything. But now I realized, keeping calm at tough times can do wonders. It took me months to be able to actually practice this!

'So you are all by yourself? It's sad that neither your mother nor mother-in-law is with you at this hour' mocked one of the typically snooty ladies I knew.

'Oh yes!', I replied sternly.

My mom, though a working woman, visited me quite frequently. Although she is claustrophobic and stays a

thousand kilometres away, she prefers the trains to flight journeys. The journey takes almost three days, but she made sure she was beside me whenever I needed her. My mom is my spine, keeping me straight and true!

During the course of my pregnancy, she had fulfilled all her duties diligently. It's just that she was not able to stay for a continuous stretch of time. But undoubtedly, she made sure she visited me along with my father once in every two months. On the other hand, my mother-in-law was still recovering from the loss of my father-in-law a few months back. She was busy completing certain official formalities and I somehow didn't want to disturb her. She made sure of phoning me whenever she could. But deep in my heart, I was sure of everyone's presence at the time of my labour.

Now this typical lady who herself was pregnant didn't bother to shut up. She knew everything about my family but rather than being sympathetic, she was being just the opposite. She would come up with statements like, 'You can take help from my aunt during your delivery, you poor lady. She knows everything and is an expert.'

I wanted to counteract by asking about her mom's arrival which didn't happen. She kept taunting me for a few more minutes and I lent her a patient ear. To my surprise, I did nothing to oppose her offensive behaviour as I would have done earlier. I had learned, 'Arguing with a fool only proves that there are two.'

I slowly left the conversation.

Back home when I shared the whole story with my husband, I just blew up. I was still mastering my patience you see!

My doctor suggested keeping myself active during the course of my pregnancy. Unlike many other pregnant women, I didn't take up pre-natal exercise classes. Rather I preferred to walk for a few minutes every day. On one hand, where my body loved being a sloth, my mind on the other asked me to be active. Usually, I would spend most of my time sitting in front of the laptop, working. Hence, I made sure I kept my body moving doing some small household chores.

I took help from my cleaning lady for completing the household chores but I didn't give up cooking. Subhashish always wanted me to keep a cook but I never agreed. For me, cooking was never a chore, it's something I loved doing. For me, cooking is therapeutic. I really cherish seeing the smile on my husband's face after a soul-filling meal. Even during my pregnancy, the thought of making a delicious breakfast or a meal made me get up from the bed. It was no longer about me or my husband, it was for our baby too! While cooking, I used to keep drinking water and have fruits to keep myself hydrated and fresh.

Salads, Curd, Fish, Chicken, Mutton, Mushroom, Assorted Lentils, Spinach and Fenugreek leaves were the items I consumed the most during my pregnancy. YouTube proved to be a boon for trying out new dishes. Pregnancy specials from Tarla Dalal and Shilpa Shetty's cookery channel were my favourites which I subscribed to for everyday healthy and delicious meals. Yes! My meals were tasty but non-spicy.

'Oh lord, the baby is kicking hard and showing its anger by pulling at the placenta', I informed my husband almost in tears. I made myself comfortably seated on a chair with the help of my husband and started rubbing my belly. I knew this was waiting to happen as I had gorged on some spicy parathas that day. I had given into the temptation of having something different and I ordered parathas stuffed with cauliflower, potato, and roasted gram flour. The tiny pieces of green chillies hidden in the stuffing couldn't be seen and they had burnt my tongue. Within no time, my eyes welled up and I could sense that I had hurt my little one inside.

I was scared to bits, sweating profusely and was really tensed about my baby but my husband comforted me by getting me a glass of water. I started cursing myself and prayed fervently to the almighty for my little one's well-being.

Neither could I hold or help the baby to stay calm. I could only communicate by rubbing my belly. 'Sorry, I'm extremely sorry. I will never hurt you again,' I kept on cajoling my baby until it stopped kicking.

After almost ten minutes, I could sense the baby being calm. I drank the remaining water and rubbed my belly apologizing and thanking it for understanding. The whole episode made me realize-

Sometimes the littlest things take up the most room in our heart.

A note from 'The soon-to-be-father':

I had said earlier that up until the time when you start to feel the baby move, it's not really real for you. Well, it was about to get real now. My wife started to 'look' pregnant now. Her belly started to protrude and she was no longer fitting into her usual dresses.

I could now feel the baby move in her belly. I could sometimes see it move as well. I started talking to the baby every night. It felt like I was really playing with the baby. It gave me immense pleasure reciting stories to the baby every night before I went to sleep.

With each passing day, I could feel my baby growing bigger. There was this amazing bond that we shared. No matter how calm and quiet the foetus remained the whole day when I was at office, every night it would start kicking and make its presence felt.

As I mentioned earlier, most of our discussions those days revolved around the baby. My wife was particularly concerned about everything she did and how it was going to affect the baby. What food she ate, what shows she watched on TV, what articles she read in the paper, what music she listened to, everything was based on how it is going to impact the baby. She would constantly keep getting advice from her mother or her aunt. The only advice I could give her about all these was 'Follow whatever the doctor says.'

13

The Baby Shower

It was a usual afternoon. After a sumptuous lunch, I lied down to take some rest when I could feel something go 'Dip! Dip! Dip!' inside my uterus. The beating was constant and kept on coming. I thought them to be the baby's kicks, albeit a lot stronger and persistent.

The baby had been with me for almost seven months now. How had I overestimated myself of knowing and gauging every movement of his? But Alas! I couldn't be more wrong.

I listened to the beats carefully but they were not the usual kicks. They were more like a continuous tapping inside my inflated belly, very similar to buzzing bumblebees. I decided to investigate for myself and scoured the internet. I read a few pages of a maternity guide and then phoned my mom. I was astounded to find out that those mild movements were actually my baby's hiccups. I slowly sipped on some water and the beats miraculously subsided after a few seconds. I was overwhelmed and had tears of joy and happiness. I had goosebumps all over. This little creature was making its presence felt with surprises every now and then. And I loved it.

Those teenie-weenie moments were making our bond stronger and drawing me closer to my little one with each passing day. We should embrace and treasure these little moments as they happen once in a lifetime. Play and converse with your baby in your own small world as I'm sure you will not get these moments back.

I couldn't wait to hold the little one in my arms. My restless mind and heart were racing against time. Just a few more months is what I say to myself!

***

It was early morning, about six when I woke up to the terrible sound of the mixer-grinder coming from the kitchen. Maybe it's a part of my dream and tried getting back to sleep. But no, it was happening for real.

Perplexed! I decided to wake up and sat in the corner of my bed. I had completely forgotten about my parents who had come to visit their expectant daughter two weeks back. Coming back to my senses, I suddenly remembered the day. It was a day of celebrations-My 'Baby Shower'.

Excited, I jumped out of the bed and headed straight towards the kitchen where I found both my parents preparing for the gala event. They had organized a small celebration and both of them wanted to make sure that each and every ritual was followed diligently. They were working as a team, preparing lunch for the guests attending the function that day.

Dad was busy helping my mom with all the grinding and the occasional stirring of the aromatic dishes. Mom, on the other hand, was the team leader. With great flair, she was multitasking- chopping, marinating the fish and getting breakfast ready simultaneously. I was not allowed to eat anything before the ritual which was supposed to commence at twelve.

It always felt great to see my parents working together and it was a joy to behold. And why not, when the whole ceremony was meant just for me? I smirked as I continued the monologue with myself.

It was around ten-thirty and it was time for me to get ready before the guests arrived. My mom draped me in an exquisite red saree and adorned me with gold accessories. Our maid, who was twice as excited as we were, brought green bangles and fresh jasmine flowers for my hair. It was such a sweet gesture!

As soon as the clock struck twelve, the guests started arriving. They brought along presents wrapped in colourful glittery papers. Few of their kids also accompanied them. Being a
traditional ritual, it became an excuse for all the moms and the elderly women to flaunt their gold-bordered saris and their antique jewellery. They all looked fabulous!

While the guests were settling down, my mom made me sit comfortably in the center, near the small shrine we had in our home. The floor was decorated with 'Rangoli' and colourful flowers. My Mom started the rituals by offering prayers to the Almighty and then doing rounds of Aarti in front of me to ward off evil. It was followed by offering me fruits which were then placed in my lap. The rest of the women followed suit. A variety of fruits- Apples, Mangoes, Pomegranate, Bananas filled my lap.

Blessings poured out of every heart. Everyone wished for my health and for a healthy baby. It was a beautiful ceremony and it meant a lot to us. But I was starving and my cravings only got stronger when the aromas from my favourite Hilsa curry filled my nostrils. It made me salivate to no end. My mom understood what I must be going through.

'Majoni, I know you must be very hungry. Just a little while more and then you can eat all you want.'

The guests were not supposed to have their lunch until I finished mine, part of the ritual! All the guests must have been waiting eagerly for me to finish eating. Poor guests, I really felt for them.

The celebration was a shift from my usual routine. Unlike other days when I used to be alone at home, busy with work, that particular day was a perfect break from the monotony. As good times pass quickly, it was time for my parents to depart. The laughter and gossip we shared was coming to an end.

'Don't worry. We might be leaving now, but will be back soon. Just take care of yourself and remember we might be far away but you are always on our minds. We love you.'

They were barely able to hold back tears as was I. A daughter always remains a child to her parents and it didn't matter if she was going to be a mom herself. With a heavy heart, I said goodbye to them until September, and wished they didn't have to go. I was emotional on seeing them go.

Next morning the house was empty again except for the two of us.

By the end of the seventh month, an intense pain due to the pressure exerted on the varicose veins left me groaning most nights. Disturbed sleep, irritated mind, painful legs all made me really uncomfortable. I couldn't lie down. All of these were the consequences of pregnancy pains, which came and went intermittently. The pain-relieving ointment and hot water leather bag came to my rescue when the pain became unbearable. Only then could I sleep in peace. Days passed by, I was about to enter the most important, the ninth month, and the thought of my delivery was making me both excited and neurotic. At times, the thought of having the baby in my arms was almost surpassed by the horrifying thoughts of being in the labour room and left me almost nauseated.

For those times, remembering these lines made me stronger and help ward off those nasty negative thoughts:

"A woman in birth is at once her most powerful and vulnerable. But any woman who has birthed unhindered understands that we are stronger than we know."

A note from 'The soon-to-be-father':

The baby shower was a family event and we had it in Bangalore. Although there were a few suggestions of organising the baby shower in our hometown, I couldn't agree with it as I thought too much travel was not a very good idea during the seventh month of pregnancy. We had our near and dear ones come to Bangalore for the event. Few rituals, some nice home cooked food and blessings from the elders were all that this little function comprised of.

The third trimester had started and these were the months of intense physical pain for the mother. She did complain of a lot of back pain, legs going numb and general tiredness. Doctor visits didn't really make a lot of difference since these pains are a part of this phase. I would try to spend more time with her and give her gentle massages and stretch her legs to alleviate the pain.

During this time, your wife will start depending upon you not only for emotional support but also physical support. There is a living person inside her. Even mundane tasks like getting up from the bed will need support. I tried to always be around. It was difficult as I had to work as well and had to be away from her for most part of the day. Setting up priorities is one thing I will recommend to all the would-be fathers at this point of time.

14

Labour & Delivery

Looking almost like a corpse, wrapped in a white sheet, I was being shifted from LDR (Labour, Delivery and Recovery) to the appointed resting room in a wheelchair.

The pain was excruciating which made me close my eyes. It took me back in time to the celebrations the evening before.

'Ladies and gentlemen, please put your hands together to welcome our next group. It's time to tap your feet to some groovy Bollywood numbers', the host announced.

Subhashish was all set to perform along with his colleagues. It was his company's Annual Day function. I accompanied him to cheer him up. The evening was well spent. We went back home late at night with the pleasurable thought of having a weekend to ourselves. We were planning a brunch together the next day. But who knew of the Almighty's plans!

At about six-thirty the next morning, I had a strong urge to pee. I went to the washroom, came back and went back to sleep. Suddenly, I developed a few minute irritable pains in my lower abdomen, I turned to the other side, calmed myself down and tried to sleep. Sleeping was hard to come by. I felt the urge to urinate again. The moment I got up, I peed on the bed. The act was involuntary. I was in shock and tried to guess what happened. Water flowed freely from my insides just like the water gushing out of a dam.

'Honey, my water broke!', I cried with astonishment. I didn't know how to react and stood still for a while.

'Don't worry, darling. It's normal in pregnancy', Subhashish replied sleepily. It had almost become a catchphrase during that time and my husband used it so often.

Though it was normal I used to fret about it.

Subhashish was still enjoying his sleep while I continued peeing on the bed.

'My water broke!' I screamed. This time he was wide awake. He jumped out of the bed with a perplexed expression on his face.

'I want to pee again. Please come with me. I'm scared', I said.

I somehow managed to get down from the bed. As soon as I sat on the commode, my legs started trembling. I was shaking with fear at the thought of my impending labour.

We were both scared, thinking that the travelling we did the day before might have had something to do with this.

'Let's go to the hospital right away', he said. 'And don't worry. Everything will be fine', he hugged me, something that I needed the most.

He put my clothes and necessary documents into a bag and I took out the sanitary pads which were unused for almost 9 months. I tried to contain the flow of the fluids with the help of the pads. In the meantime, Subhashish called for a cab. The cab came within no time and we left for the hospital.

We must have been in the car only for a few minutes when a black cat crossed our way. My mind started racing because of the superstitions associated with black cats crossing paths.

I felt sad and sensing that my driver stopped the car. It was a bad omen, superstitious beliefs, you know!

Subhashish sensed the turbulent thoughts in my mind. He cracked a joke that forced me to laugh. But deep down, my heart was pounding. I knew even his mind was not at peace but who else could be my spine if he broke down? And he knew that!

It was around eight in the morning when we reached the hospital. I managed to walk just barely as the water continued to leak.

'My wife's water broke, please suggest which way to go', Subhashish asked the receptionist. The receptionist informed us that we should head to the LDR room.

'Madam, can I get you a wheelchair?', the receptionist asked me.

'No thanks, I'm fine!' I replied.

On reaching the LDR, I was asked to lie down on the bed. The nurse was informed of the water break. She asked me to change my dress and gave me a pink apron to wear. She then tied my big belly with a stretchable belt, asked me to hold an indicator which was connected to a reading machine. The machine was reading my contractions and my baby's heartbeat. Subhashish sat on the stool next to me and started informing our parents.

At around eight-thirty, one of the junior doctors stepped in. She was of medium height, young, her long hair beautifully plaited. She had sharp facial features and a shrill voice. She stormed inside and put on disposable gloves.

'I need to do an internal examination', she informed me and asked my husband to leave the room until called.

The nurse smeared some gel on her fingers and Oh! Lord! I screamed. I bit my fingers to endure the pain as the junior doctor inserted her fingers mercilessly. She pushed her fingers as much as she could.

'What are you doing? Put your butt down', she yelled at me. Her frustrated and irritated voice made me want to kick her away from my bed.

'She is 2 centimetres dilated', she informed the nurse and my husband as soon he was called in.

'She is not getting either the pains or the contractions. We need to monitor her for another hour. If she still doesn't get pains we will have to induce it', she added. In the meantime, I was served breakfast and was instructed to press the indicator whenever the contractions arose. After about an hour, the nurse reported that the heart rate of our baby was healthy and there was an improvement in the contractions. However, the pains I was experiencing were minimal and hence it was decided to get them induced. The nurse fitted the cannula into my left hand, near the thumb and injected me with an IV drug that flowed all the way to my vagina.

The junior doctor came into the room, checked the readings-my contractions and the baby's heart rate. She wanted my blood and urine samples. She left the room at about one.

The nurse on duty took my blood and sent it for testing. They were running various tests on me and the reading machine was monitoring my contractions. Subhashish, who was sitting by my side, kept on encouraging me as I was confused and tensed about undergoing labour.

'Ah! I'm getting the pains, I'm getting the pains', I screamed as I held Subhashish's hand. The pains would come for a few seconds and then vanish. The contractions started to happen every 15 minutes, then 10minutes, then 5 minutes and so on during the labour. My husband's eyes were focused on the graphs on the reading machine monitor. I was pacing the room, sometimes talking and sometimes resting.

As the clock struck one, it was time for the brute to enter, the junior doctor. As soon as she entered the room, she asked my husband to leave the room. She got ready with her gloves on and with the gel smeared on her fingers.

'Please do it slowly this time', I almost begged.

'When you come to the hospital you have to expect some pain, dear', she answered in her merciless tone with a cunning smile on her lips. While going through the examination this time, I remembered my practitioner, Dr. Suman Singh's advice- take long deep breaths while slowly moving down your butt. She removed her fingers from my vagina and announced that I was 4 centimetres dilated. The junior doctor asked the nurse to serve me lunch followed by the enema dose. Hot khichdi was served. I was not able to eat due to the irritating contractions.

'Please eat. You will definitely need the energy and strength now', one of the nurses advised. My husband fed me and somehow I was able to finish my lunch. We shared the meal as I was afraid of him leaving me alone in the LDR.

And finally, Dr. Suman showed up. She saw the reports and informed that the delivery could be expected anywhere between eight and nine that night. The enema was done and I was kept on a liquid diet thereafter.

From the other room, I could hear another woman undergoing labour. She was moaning with pain. Her painful screams were frightening me. The nurses decided to shift me to the resting room that was appointed for me.

'Please keep your feet down on the foot-plates', one of the nurses assisted me. Suddenly I came back to reality. I could barely open my eyelids. I was then transferred to a bed and attached to a monitor. My husband was sitting next to me and saw the immense increase in the contractions. The pain was intense and the moment it heightened I used to squeeze his palms. I was shifted to another room from the LDR as by then we knew that the delivery might get delayed.

One of the junior doctors stepped in. Thankfully, she was not the one who showed up in the morning. Unlike the previous one, this doctor was gentle and polite. She wanted to check the progress of my dilation, she put on her gloves and applied the gel on top of her fingers and then inserted her fingers. It was gentler than the earlier one. The clean white gloves came out red.

Her face gave a surprised look. 'She is 8cms dilated!', exclaimed the junior doctor. It was a surprise to everyone in the room as it was around four in the afternoon and the delivery wasn't expected until about nine that night. 'Doctor, she is full', she phoned Dr. Singh.

Dr. Singh who had finished her duty and was home by that time came running to my rescue. I was instructed to shift to the LDR again and was made to sit in the wheelchair. As soon as I was about to sit, I was seized by contractions. I asked them to wait until the contractions ceased. After that, I was transferred to the LDR within no time. I was followed by two of the nurses with my husband walking by my side.

The once silent LDR room turned into the busiest room with many nurses in action. Few were helping me get into the correct position and the others were busy keeping the medical instruments ready for the delivery of the baby.

No doubt I was nervous and scared, however, the junior doctor was trying to divert my mind as they asked Subhashish to step out of the room. I started chanting and praying to the Almighty. A few minutes later, Dr. Suman Singh came and both the doctors quickly wore their green scrubs and caps. The nurses rearranged the sides of the bed to adjust two horizontal stands to rest my feet on. My legs were wide open and Dr. Singh sat in between them. To her left was the trolley with steel bowls that contained scissors, knives and what not! The junior doctor stood by Dr. Singh's side. On her right, the nurses were standing by to help Dr. Singh during the process. I was asked to hold my big thighs and to exert pressure while pushing. Dr. Singh was kind enough to summon my husband in. On my left stood one of the nurses pressing my belly gently in order to help push my baby and Subhashish gently rubbing my back.

'Take long breaths and push it harder when contractions happen', advised Dr. Singh. I tried pushing, closed my eyes and roared but in vain.

'Don't make sounds but use the energy to push the baby', the nurse suggested while pressing my belly. I tried but failed. Dr. Singh instructed me again and this time I did it. I pushed it with such a force that I felt something burst out from my body.

Owah....Owah... I could hear the feeble cries of my baby and

Boy! Was I relieved! Overwhelmed, tears flowed down my cheeks but I was smiling. I don't know how to express that feeling. Moments such as these can never be put into words. Words can never do justice to the intensely sensational feelings I was going through. Subhashish and I both glanced at each other, congratulating each other on finally becoming parents. What a journey we have had and we were holding the culmination in our arms. Everyone in the room congratulated us. Dr. Singh and the junior doctor closed the incision which they had made to take the baby out. We were so excited that we had completely forgotten to ask whether it was a boy or a girl. We were just happy and content that we gave birth a beautiful soul- healthy and happy and the gender did not matter.

'It's a boy!' exclaimed one of the nurses.

The nurses cleaned and brought our baby to us. We couldn't believe we were holding our baby. We were so over the moon that the thought of capturing the moment completely slipped off our minds. A nurse was kind enough to click a picture of the three of us. I kept admiring my baby and I couldn't believe my eyes that the little creature that had just been born was inside me all those nine months.

We three spent some time together. After a few minutes, they took the baby and put it in a cradle to rest. Subhashish went out of the room and made a few calls informing everyone about the good news.

'My nipples are paining, can you please increase the temperature?', I asked one of the staff in the room. Even though she increased the temperature of the AC, the pain didn't go away.

'Feed your baby, you will feel better', one of the nurses advised.

She came holding my baby and gave it to me. The moment I held him, I felt exhilarated. At the same time, I was baffled about the correct way to feed him. The nurse helped both of us with the proper way of feeding. Breastfeeding is the best feeling, I must say! And whoa! the pain subsided.

After the feeding was done, the baby was then shifted to his room and I was asked to take a bath. I cleaned the blood stains and the nurse helped me in scrubbing my body. The warm water skimmed off all the weariness from my body. Finally, both my baby and I shifted to our appointed resting room.

Both of our parents came down to Bangalore and reached the hospital. Everyone wished us and blessed our baby. For the next two days, room number 106 became my home. I was resting, feeding, eating and welcoming the guests in to our room.

Finally, the time came when our little baby was about to start for his little abode. Everything felt like part of a fairy tale. From there on, the journey was not at all an easy one but it was indeed very interesting. As I believe, *"Challenges are what make life interesting; overcoming them is what makes life meaningful"*.

As new parents, we were celebrating this new bond with our baby with a belief that God has trusted us with this precious gift and he will guide us as we embark on yet another fantastic journey.

A note from 'The Father':

We just had our office annual day function. It was late. I was a little drunk and very tired. We were returning home in a cab at around midnight. On our way I said to my wife, 'Good that we have a weekend coming up. I need to sleep till afternoon tomorrow.'

Early next morning, I wake up to the words, 'I think my water broke.' I was having a hangover. She had given me many false alarms before. I didn't give much attention to her at first. But soon she told me again that it seemed her water had indeed broken this time. I woke up to find the bed all wet. I held her and took her to the washroom. I booked a cab immediately and told her that we were going to the hospital.

The function was at a place that was quite far from our home. We travelled the distance in a cab. Bangalore roads are not as smooth as you want a major metropolitan to have. I was skeptical that the bumpy road might have caused her health to go bad all of a sudden. The delivery due date was still two weeks away. I was nervous and was cursing myself for going out for a party when my wife is nine months pregnant.

After the initial diagnosis, the nurse came out and told me, 'The water bag has broken. We will get the baby delivered today. We will get her admitted.'

I started breathing easy now. She was in the hospital now, there was nothing to worry about. Doctors were there to take care of her. I started making some phone calls to let my family and friends know. The doctors said we would have to wait for some time as the labor pain had not started yet. I was with my wife while the pain was increasing. She held my hand and squeezed it really hard when the contractions began.

It was almost evening when she was transferred to the labor room for delivery. I was there along with her. After about half an hour, I was able to see the baby coming out. It was around six-thirty in the evening when our baby boy saw the world for the first time. I cut the umbilical cord myself. Soon, I was holding the tiny life form in my arms. I went to my wife, she held him close. This was the moment we had been waiting for and it was no less magical than we had imagined it to be.

The Journey Continues...

Our son is going to complete four years this September and here we are still figuring it out. Is it happening for real? All these months have passed by but we are still finding it hard to believe that we gave birth to this beautiful soul who has brightened our lives with his infectious smile and naughty antics.

Sometimes I go back in time and find myself standing in the basketball court of our school waiting for Subhashish, just to speak a few words. Never in our wildest dreams could we have thought that we would come this far. We met for the first time in October, 2002. Eyes met, feelings exchanged and we ended up becoming soul mates. Good times, bad times- we have seen it all. Beautiful moments made us grateful and the bad ones made us strong. Long distance relationships, reunions, separations-all were part of this journey. Given a chance, I'll do it all over again. As teenagers, we travelled together holding hands, grew up together as adults and are blessed as parents now.

This pregnancy has made our bond stronger than ever before. We are thankful to the universe for bringing us together and answering our wishes and prayers with Lakshya.

Testimonials

"Choosing to have a baby is said to be a life-defining decision as it bears an irrevocable impact on the mother, physically and psychologically. You not just carry a life within but grow with it, too.

Banani's book 'Emotions & Elation' is a beautiful compilation of these changes during her pregnancy and how beautifully she embraces them all! Unlike any pregnancy guide or manual, the book has her personal moments and experiences that makes it exquisite. Adding another angle to the book is the involvement of her husband who shoulders THEIR pregnancy throughout the 9-months and is open about sharing the responsibilities. That is a welcome change considering not many men are comfortable talking about the birth of their child and it remains to be a mother's prerogative.

The book is beautifully crafted with her emotions."

Richa Saxena

Social Media Strategist &
Mommy Blogger

“Nothing can be as pure and serene as words coming straight from a mom’s heart. I really look forward to this book of Banani expressing a million emotions a would be mom and even dad go thorough as they welcome their precious piece of heart into the world.”

Roma Gupta Sinha
Author

"An engaging read, this book took me on a gentle trip down the memory lane when I was expecting my son. Pregnancy brings you closer as a couple, and Banani and Shubhashish's journey is a proof of that."

Ghazal Alagh
Founder-Mamaearth

A Note on the Author

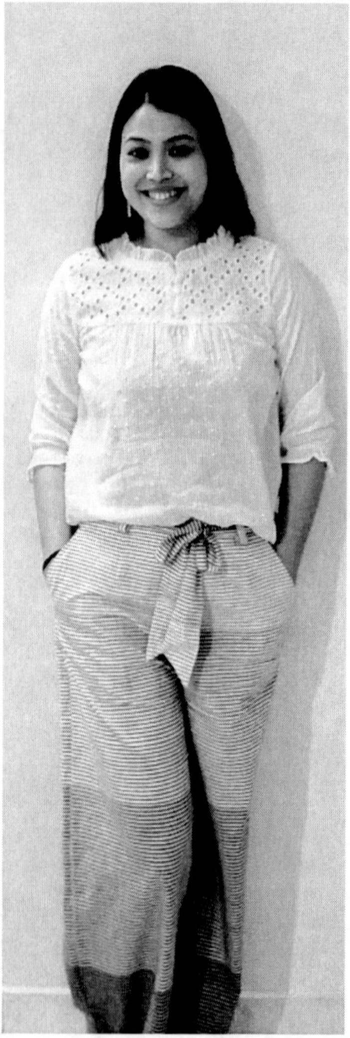

Banani Das Dhar, an ex-clinical data analyst turned entrepreneur, founder- BananiVista, a knowledge sharing platform.

She is an Author (Emotions & Elation), Educator, Bharatnatyam Dancer, Mindfulness Practitioner, Dance Meditation teacher & a Youth Mental Health Influencer.

Awarded by MSME World in appreciation of achievement in Entrepreneurship.

Banani believes in the saying, "The secret to growth is helping others grow." Since 2014, through her blog (now turned a knowledge-sharing forum, Banani has been consistently working towards inspiring, transforming & empowering people. She conducts a variety of workshops for both kids & adults and help them finding their voice.

Banani's work has been published in prestigious newspapers, magazines & journals, being Femina, The Bold Outline, Deccan Herrald & The New Indian Express to name a few.

Banani through her organization has also conducted philanthropic activities for various NGO's. She is looking to collaborate with more such organizations to give back to the universe.

Apart from following her passion for writing, the author is an avid traveler too. She has always considered herself an explorer, with a zeal and passion to find out more. For her, traveling is not just a way to discover new places, it also gives her an opportunity to self-reflect. It becomes a path to self-discovery. Combining these two gifts she tries to bring her varied experiences to create a vivid imagery in the minds of her audience.

Her ever so willing partner in crime is her husband, who has staunchly stood by her wishes. They have been together for more than fifteen years now and they complete each other in every way. They hope to create many more fabulous memories with their bundle of joy- Lakshya too!

Although this is the author's debut book, she has contributed to numerous anthologies. She loves penning down both fictional and non-fictional stories.

She can be reached at bananivista2017@gmail.com